Living With a Stranger

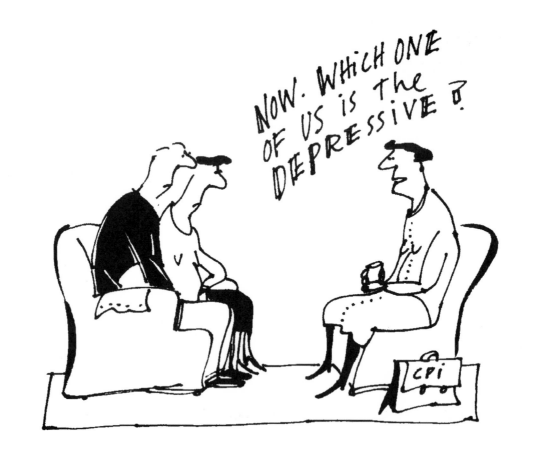

By VALERIE STILLWELL

Drawings by Christine Roche

Living With a Stranger

GASKELL/WEST LONDON HEALTH PROMOTION AGENCY

Text © The Royal College of Psychiatrists 1997
Drawings © Christine Roche 1997

Gaskell is an imprint of the Royal College of Psychiatrists,
17 Belgrave Square, London SW1X 8PG

British Library Cataloguing-in-Publication Data
A catalogue record for this book is available from the British Library.

ISBN 1-901242-07-2

Distributed in North America
by American Psychiatric Press, Inc.
ISBN 0-88048-582-5

Printed in Great Britain by Bell & Bain Ltd, Glasgow.

Contents

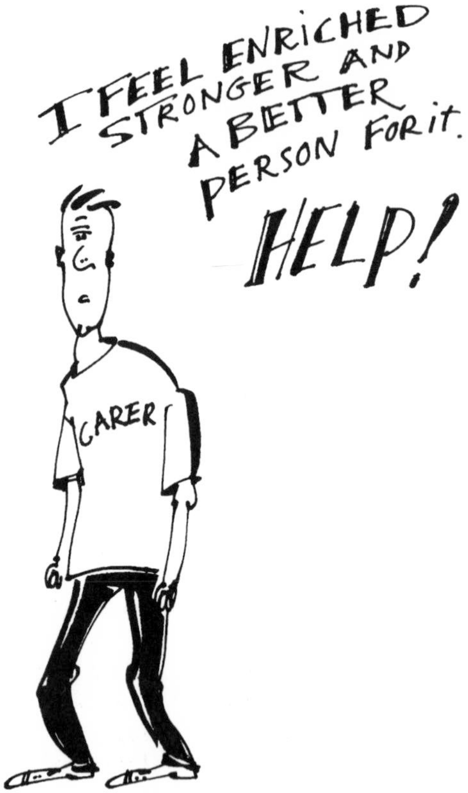
I FEEL ENRICHED STRONGER AND A BETTER PERSON FOR it.
HELP!
CARER

Foreword

Depression is a common and often severe disorder. Although estimates vary, up to 50% of women and 25% of men will suffer from depression at some time during their lives. Research also shows that depression is common in teenagers, and can even occur in young children. Unfortunately, depression tends to come back, with the majority of depressed people suffering from an episodic, recurring illness.

Depression is associated with a number of physical illnesses, and an increased risk of suicide. The physical, psychological, social and work-related problems linked with depression appear to be greater than those seen in some physical illnesses, including arthritis, high blood pressure and diabetes. For example, the early development of children can be slowed down by postnatal depression in the mother. Depression also reduces quality of life, can interfere with family relationships and may have devastating effects on financial income.

Although common, depression is sometimes difficult to recognise. Unfortunately there is still a stigma attached to depression, and many people worry that talking about their feelings will lead to problems at home or at work. Research shows that most people with depression do visit their family doctor, but not necessarily with symptoms of depression. Recognition is sometimes difficult because of the reluctance of patients and doctors to discuss emotional problems, the tendency for patients to start consultations with physical symptoms, and the short time that is available for consultation in many health care settings.

Research also shows that doctors differ in their attitude to depressed patients, some regarding it as an interesting challenge, but others feeling uncomfortable with psychological problems and believing that treating depressed patients can be rather unrewarding. Of the depressed people who seek help from their family doctors, many are not recognised as suffering from depression, at least not at first. Even when patients are diagnosed as depressed, the treatment they receive from their doctor can be inadequate.

All this may make depressing reading! This would be particularly unfortunate, as depression is a very treatable condition. Many treatments are available, and when used appropriately can not only relieve depressive symptoms but also reduce the difficulties associated with depression. For example, antidepressant drugs are clearly effective in the treatment of patients with depressive symptoms of at least moderate severity, and antidepressants have also been found effective in long-term treatment, designed to prevent a relapse or recurrence of depression. In addition, psychological therapies (talking treatments) such as cognitive therapy and interpersonal therapy have been found helpful in both short- and long-term treatment, and may enhance the benefits of antidepressant drugs.

So, depression is common, serious and treatable, but often missed. For these reasons, the UK Defeat Depression Campaign was launched in January 1992. Organised by the Royal College of Psychiatrists, in association with the Royal College of General Practitioners, the Campaign was a five-year initiative designed to assist health care professionals in the recognition and treatment of patients with depressive illness, and to increase public understanding of the nature, course and treatment of depression. Preliminary findings show that the Campaign may have contributed to positive changes in public awareness and understanding of depression; its effects on professional practice are currently being evaluated.

The Defeat Depression Campaign came to its formal end in December 1996. However, there is a clear need for further similar activities, as producing beneficial changes in the understanding and management of depression is likely to be a long-term task. In part, this will be helped by improved teaching of medical students and the continuous education of doctors and other health professionals.

Some of the needs of depressed people remain unmet, even with effective drug treatments and psychological therapies. Self-help and mutual support also play a significant role. Through local groups and a central office, the self-help organisation Depression Alliance provides support, advice and information for depressed people, while also seeking to improve public awareness and encourage research. The defeat of depression requires more than just professional development. Further public education is required to address and minimise the stigma of depression. Books such as this play an important role in improving public understanding of depression, and can complement the benefits of other forms of treatment, thereby increasing the chances of lasting recovery.

David S. Baldwin

Senior Lecturer in Psychiatry, University of Southampton; Member of the Defeat Depression Campaign Management Committee 1991–1996; President of Depression Alliance

Preface

I had no idea what lay ahead when my husband, Peter, became depressed and I could not find a book that answered my needs, though there were plenty written about depression itself. What I wanted was a sort of rough guide as to what to expect and how to cope. *Living With a Stranger* is written for others who find themselves in a similar situation. Although depression is more common in women than men, I have written from a wife's point of view and I hope you will overlook the use of the male gender throughout.

I coped because I had to. In my case it was a complete role reversal from dependant wife to breadwinner and somewhat assertive female. It has done me a power of good, though I can't speak for the rest of the family!

I learned all I could about depression in order to find out what I was up against, but nothing had prepared me for the bewildering emotions I would experience and which were, I now think, quite natural in the circumstances.

Two things stand out as being of particular help to me. A friend whose close relative had been through a depressive illness gave me a time-scale. Within a year, he said, Peter would be back at work, and by the end of 18 months he would be 80% well again. This gave me something to look forward to.

The other thing that helped was when I was eventually able to tell people what was wrong with Peter and why. We received a great deal of sympathy and support from everyone and it was surprising the number of people who knew about depression, sometimes at first hand. It was a relief to be able to talk about it and share the problem.

Additionally, our three children were incredibly supportive, each in their own way.

Five years on I have never known Peter to be so well, cheerful and confident, and our relationship has been enriched by our experience.

May you, too, have your happy ending.

Valerie Stillwell

Introduction

When you consider that 5% of the population suffers from depression at any one time, then you could probably assume that another 5% or more must be affected by it too – their close family and friends.

It is not easy living with a depressed person. The strain on relationships can be enormous, at times overwhelming. You, as the carer, are vulnerable.

Yet your role is very important. A positive attitude to your partner's illness is vital for their swift recovery and the prevention of future bouts of depression. You are their lifeline back to wholeness and health.

How are you to cope with the change in the person you love? How can you help them? How are you to manage your own feelings and at the same time get the others around you safely through this distressing time?

There are ways of coping. A depressed person *will* get better and you will find that this life-disrupting illness can lead to a deeper relationship between you.

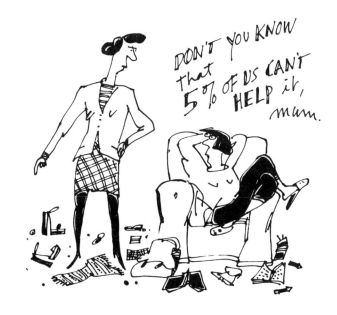

1 Recognising depression

Most of us get depressed at times, but true depression, or clinical depression, is an actual illness. It is so widespread that it has become known as 'the common cold of mental illness'.

You are probably the first person to see the change in your partner. At work, or with friends, they 'cover up'. Gradually, though, the illness takes over. A formerly cheerful outgoing man becomes withdrawn and morose. An attractive caring woman will neglect her appearance and relationships, becoming completely absorbed in self-misery. To those close to them, it really is like living with a stranger.

What is this illness?

The word depression means being pushed or pressed down. It is more than just a low mood, a feeling of dejection or an attack of 'the blues'. It can affect anyone of any age or background, but is greatly misunderstood by the general public. Depression is not a state of mind or a character weakness; it is a recognised clinical illness.

Research into the causes and treatment of depression focus on biochemical changes in the brain. Two neurotransmitters (these are chemical 'messengers' in the brain) called noradrenaline and serotonin are involved. In a depressed person their activity is reduced, but it returns to normal once they recover.

A form of depression outside my experience and not discussed here is manic depression, in which a person has extreme 'highs' of great energy and elation, followed by 'lows' of utter lethargy and despair.

Signs and symptoms

The form which depression takes can vary, but there are certain symptoms which are characteristic:

- loss of concentration
- feelings of sadness and a tendency to cry
- becoming withdrawn
- preoccupation with negative thoughts
- self-blame
- extreme exhaustion
- loss of interest in life
- lack of motivation
- unreliability
- loss of self-confidence
- lack of interest in sex
- over- or under-eating
- excessive drinking
- change in sleeping pattern
- mixed-up thoughts
- physical aches and pains
- restlessness
- anxiety and possibly suicidal feelings.

Any of these may be experienced, plus irrational fears and phobias. A daunting list. But the good news is that depression is almost always curable and

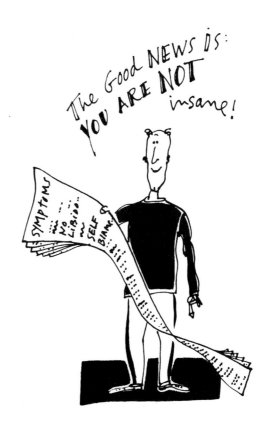

where it is not the symptoms can be relieved to a great extent.

Looking at the causes

There is no single cause of clinical depression, although a traumatic event such as bereavement or job loss may trigger it off in someone who is vulnerable. What happened to someone as a child can have an effect on how they react later on. It may have helped shape their self-image, their ability to love and feel loved or feel wanted – their attitude to life.

However, there are some events which are recognised as stress factors. Should a person experience two or more such events within a short period of time, this could lead to a bout of depression.

Depression is also more likely to happen at certain times of life, such as puberty, new parenthood, menopause and retirement.

Statistically, women are more likely to suffer from depression than men. There could be several reasons for this. Women may be more willing to seek help than men who may try to hide the symptoms, possibly by drinking. There may be genetic or hormonal reasons, premenstrual syndrome and menopause. Postnatal depression can occur after the birth of a baby and may last weeks, months or even years if untreated. Mothers with several small children and an unsupportive or absent partner are vulnerable, particularly if their living conditions are poor. Married women, apparently, suffer the illness more than married men.

Other more obvious causes are:

- loneliness
- bereavement
- marriage problems or divorce
- unemployment or redundancy
- financial difficulties
- moving house
- work overload or failure to obtain promotion
- prolonged strain, such as nursing someone who is disabled in some way
- severe shock
- imprisonment
- having experienced incest or other traumas as a child.

In Peter's case there were several factors leading up to his illness. We had spent most of our married

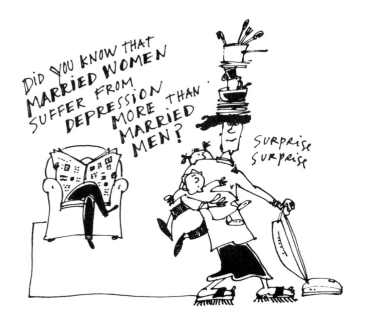

DID YOU KNOW THAT MARRIED WOMEN SUFFER FROM DEPRESSION MORE THAN MARRIED MEN?

SURPRISE SURPRISE

life in South Africa, where he was brought up. His mother had suffered a series of strokes and was no longer the cheerful person we knew. When his father died a year or so later, Peter had difficulty coming to terms with it. To make things worse, I was constantly homesick for the UK.

Unexpectedly, there was a job offer from England and he accepted it, suggesting we give it a two-year trial, but moving house, changing jobs and country was a recipe for disaster. After only a year in England, during which time we moved house three more times, he became deeply depressed and consequently lost his job.

What the sufferer feels

A depressed person has an extremely negative attitude to everything. The glass is never half full, it is always half empty. Life seems pointless. They think they are bad and worthless and there is no hope for them. Does all this strike a chord?

The other side of depression, which can be difficult to understand if you've never experienced it, is the feeling of utter isolation. No one else can know what

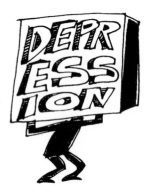

they are going through, no one else can be 'in there' with them. Sufferers have described depression as 'being at the bottom of a deep, dark pit', 'trapped in a thick, choking smog', or 'like being in hell'.

They are experiencing a mental pain which is as bad as, or worse than, physical pain. You cannot see it, but then you cannot see an earache or a migraine. (Patients who deliberately hurt themselves physically, often by cutting their arms, say that it gives them a visible pain to focus on for a while, taking their attention away from the inner agony.)

How long, you may wonder, does it all last? If I say it takes approximately 18 months for someone to be cured, that might sound pessimistic. But depression takes its own time to work itself out, and there may be minor setbacks along the road to recovery. However, they will be functioning well long before then, back at work in all probability, and they should be themselves again by the end of 18 months. Also, strange as it sounds, you can both benefit from the experience.

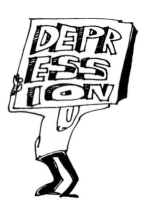

2 Taking a positive approach

Being there

It is hard work being around a depressed person but, difficult or not, your presence is very important. A depressed person's most common fear is that of being alone. Simply by being there you are helping, even though he appears to ignore you much of the time. Your presence is reassuring. It shows that you care, that you love him, and that is what a depressed person needs most.

Often it will feel as though you are talking to a brick wall. He does not communicate or respond, unless it is to voice a negative thought.

'I don't know why you bother, I'm not worth it. If I were dead you'd be better off.'

He may have irrational fears, worries that are exaggerated out of all proportion, For instance he may be frightened to drive his car, even though he has been driving for 20 years and it is second nature

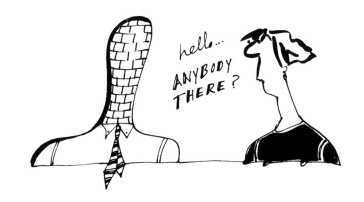

to him. He may have fears of being thrown out onto the streets, of ending up destitute. He may express a fear of going mad or even dying – 'You don't understand, I'm not going to live through this, I'm going to die.'

This is a deeply depressed person speaking, totally absorbed in his misery. If your relative is down in the trough of depression you will hear similar fears expressed over and over again. Each time you must counteract them, biting your tongue, counting to ten. Just keep on reassuring him. To the ill person his fears are very real. He wants his pain to end and he doesn't want his family to suffer. Death seems to be the only solution. Your presence, though, puts the brakes on. Perhaps it even gives him a glimmer of hope.

Finding help

Of course, you can't be there all the time. The daily routine has to go on as normally as possible. The children have to be taken to school, shopping has to be bought, visits to the dentist or library made. You have your own job or career to consider. You may have to take a full-time job to supplement the family income while your partner is ill. What happens then?

This is where family, friends, neighbours and the social services come in. You need sitters, people who can take over or call in regularly when you are not there. A relative may offer to live with you temporarily and act as a carer. A rota of sitters/visitors can be drawn up so you can be sure there are one or two friendly faces calling in each day. You should also leave a list of telephone numbers handy, including your work number, your general practitioner's (GP's) and those of the community psychiatric nurse (CPN) and social services. If you have a dependable neighbour who is able to pop in every so often to check everything is all right, you could give them a door key.

In the early stages of the illness it could benefit your partner if they are able to talk to someone. It could prevent the illness from becoming life-disrupting or even life-threatening. It may give them a chance to change their lifestyle before it pushes them under; for example, finding a less stressful job, or having bereavement counselling.

In an ideal society many different talking treatments would be available, and the user would be able to choose a therapist with whom they felt a rapport, someone to listen, understand, care and help rebuild their confidence. Sadly, this is not yet an option, but

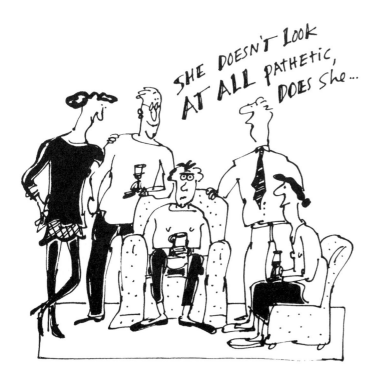

SHE DOESN'T LOOK AT ALL PATHETIC, DOES SHE...

hopefully it will be in the future. Many GPs, CPNs and social workers have training in counselling, and talking with them can be valuable. Your local MIND group may also have counsellors available. Private counsellors and psychotherapists are available if you can afford them. National Health Service counsellors, usually based at GP surgeries, often have a lengthy waiting list.

The CPN will visit you at home and listen to both your partner's and your own problems and help you reach a solution. Social workers also offer support and practical advice. They provide information on other services which may be of use to you. For example, they can put you in touch with a local support group for depressed people and relatives if there is one. They can also organise a home care assistant (home help) or meals on wheels if necessary. They help and advise on most personal and financial problems.

Forms of support from the social services vary from district to district. Make use of them; they are there for you.

The Citizens' Advice Bureau and the Samaritans are among other organisations that are there for you. Take any help that is offered. Don't be afraid or too proud to ask.

Your GP may refer the patient to a consultant at the local hospital. Yes – the psychiatrist. Now, before you run a mile, think it over. There should be no shame or embarrassment in consulting a psychiatrist. They are doctors who specialise, just as neurologists or paediatricians do. Their speciality is mental illness as opposed to physical illness. They will discuss the patient's problems, prescribe treatment, or in very severe cases suggest a stay in hospital.

What not to do

Without wishing to contradict the positive attitude in the title of this chapter, I would like to suggest a few things you should avoid when you are with a depressed person.

There is a fine line between keeping cheerful – which is essential for everyone's sake – and being insensitively over-cheerful. In other words, jollying him along, telling him to cheer-up and pull himself together. He *cannot*. That is what the illness is all about, so however tempted you may be to utter the words – don't. He no longer has the energy to try. Urging him to do so hurts because he thinks you are blaming him for his condition, criticising behaviour which is entirely beyond his control.

By telling him to get his act together you are only adding to his burden of guilt and self-hatred. He is unable to look on the bright side because from where he is standing there isn't one.

It does not help to point out that there are others who are worse off, either. I have heard depressed people say 'I know there are people starving and dying of cancer and AIDS, but that doesn't help me. I am in hell.'

It goes without saying that you should not criticise or reproach him, but you may find it difficult not to argue with him. You can empathise with his self-pity, for instance, but you should not condone or condemn it. You must not reinforce his negativity. It is better simply to stick to positive statements, such as 'I know that you are suffering and I can't imagine what it must be like, but I *do* know that you will come through it eventually.'

However irritated you are with the constant repetition of negative thoughts, try to switch off. Do your best to hide your anger and frustration when you are with them. It is hard, I know. Keep biting your tongue!

Making things easier

When you are around there are practical ways in which you can make time pass more easily for the patient.

Make a list of small jobs that need doing around the house or garden, a bit of DIY or weeding. You must not have expectations that are too high, though, or he will feel pressured or inadequate if he finds he cannot manage them. And no nagging! Praise any achievements, however small. To a depressed person it has taken an enormous amount of effort. The important thing is to get through each day as best you (both) can, leaving him little time to sit and brood.

Involve him in a hobby if he has the energy, but be prepared for him to say that he can't concentrate. Inability to concentrate is a feature of depression.

Daily walks and gentle exercise are important. Spectator sports, gardening, painting (both kinds, art and interior decorating) are therapeutic. A change of scenery is often welcome, and pets can be a blessing. Watching a moving or uplifting play, film or concert on television can release emotions (yours as well as his), which can be a relief.

In a depressed state a person does not think life is worth getting up for in the morning, so he will need encouragement. It is often in the mornings that they are at their lowest.

Being so absorbed with his inner misery and mental pain he may ignore his appearance and personal cleanliness. Coax him to have a shower or bath daily, shave himself and put on fresh clothes. He probably won't do so otherwise, and will slop around in his oldest clothes for days, unkempt, and with lank, greasy hair. Later, when he is recovering, he will be glad that you encouraged him to attend to his personal appearance and helped preserve his dignity.

At meal times offer him a plate of food even though he says he is not hungry and picks at the food. He may well have lost weight, but he will put it on again when he gets better. He might prefer a meal supplement such as Complan or Fortisip. Caffeine and alcohol are both depressants, so limit their intake, or stop using them altogether. If your GP has prescribed antidepressants for him, he will already have been warned not to drink alcohol.

At some point, when you judge it to be the right time, you could sit down with him and write a list of his main worries and problems. Help him out by

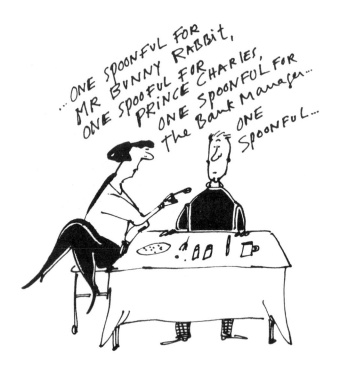

...ONE SPOONFUL FOR MR BUNNY RABBIT, ONE SPOONFUL FOR PRINCE CHARLES, ONE SPOONFUL FOR the Bank Manager... ONE SPOONFUL...

asking leading questions, otherwise he may shrug and tell you it is 'everything'. Some problems may be imaginary – 'I'll never be able to drive my car again'. He will.

Other problems may be real. He could, for instance, have lost his job. Face the problems one at a time and see what can be done to alleviate or overcome them. Work out what will need to be changed in your lives in order to deal with the depression. If there is something wrong with your relationship, contact Relate for counselling, either then or when he is coming out of the depression.

If he has suffered a loss of some kind, he will need bereavement counselling. When you confront problems, always get professional help if you feel out of your depth.

Aromatherapy and massage have been found to be therapeutic by many sufferers. You could teach yourself a few massage strokes to use on your partner. Massage could help you, too. After all, you are also in a stressful situation.

Read up all you can about depression. The more you understand this painful illness the better. Just keep remembering that people don't want to be depressed and they cannot help the way they behave.

Keep reinforcing the idea that it is a temporary condition and he will get better in time. Touch him, hug him, listen to him and even cry with him if it comes to it. Forget all that stiff-upper-lip bit. Crying can be good for you. Bolster his ego by reminding him of his successes in the past. Talk of future aims and goals. This is all therapy for him. It is part of the purpose of your being there. It also shows that you love him.

Responsibilities

When one member of a family or partnership is ill, some of their responsibilities fall on others. A wife who formerly left the finances in her husband's hands will have to pay the bills. If the couple has a joint account it is straightforward, but if not she might have to contact a solicitor to obtain power of attorney in order to sign cheques and other documents on her husband's behalf. She may also need help filling in income tax returns if her husband had previously done it. Money, or the lack of it, can be an added burden, so, once again, get professional help.

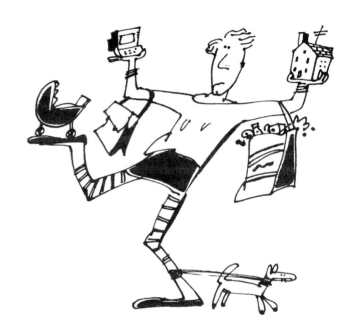

It was quite a shock to my system realising I had to take charge of the household finances. Most of our money was still tied up in South Africa at the time so I had to take on a full-time job to support us. Ironically, the only one available was in a psychiatric hospital!

A man may find himself thrust into the role of house-husband, responsible for housekeeping and looking after the children. Other responsibilities can be delegated to different members of the family. Everyday things like cooking, laundry and cleaning can be shared tasks.

Depression can be infectious, so be good to yourselves. Let the children stay over with their friends and vice versa. Take the family to a theme park, or go to a theatre or concert. A few little treats now and then cheer everyone up.

Decision-making

Many of the decisions a carer makes are minor ones, such as urging the depressed person to visit the doctor. He may be reluctant to go because there is 'nothing to see'. Make the appointment yourself and accompany him. Make sure he takes any medication the GP prescribes.

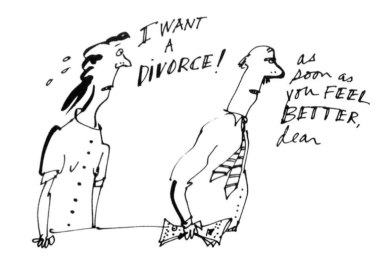

If he is running out of sick leave and in danger of losing his job, you could visit his employers and explain the situation. It is possible they can come to some arrangement whereby they can hold the job over for a certain period, or ease him back in with part-time employment when he shows signs of improvement.

It is very important that you do not allow a depressed person to make any major life-changing decisions. The illness exaggerates his thinking and puts him in a state of panic. He could make decisions that are not appropriate. Giving in his notice, for instance, or putting the house on the market. Divorce is another major decision he might contemplate. (This is quite common among depressives. It is another form of 'you'd be better off without me'.) Try and diffuse the situation. Explain that all big decisions must be left until he is well.

If there is any basis for these, albeit exaggerated, fears, now could be the time for you to face them. Is he struggling in his job? Would he be happier living somewhere else? Do you have problems in your relationship? Think them over. Dismiss them if they are nonsense, but bear in mind that later on you may need professional help in reaching important decisions.

3 Making everyday life normal

As a carer, your daily life will to a certain extent revolve round the patient. You have to take care that you do not cut short the time and attention you give to the rest of the family. They need support too. It is no fun having the dampening effect of a depressed person around. The mood can take over. Try and keep the atmosphere as light and cheerful as possible.

In milder forms of depression the sufferer may become irritable and intolerant, giving way to outbursts of anger over things which would not normally bother them. They become sensitive to everyday noises; the radio, children's chatter, the sound of the washing machine. These outbursts, which seem to be for no reason, are upsetting to the household, causing friction and souring of relationships. Irritability has a tendency to 'rub off' on others.

However, remember that it *is* a symptom and therefore temporary.

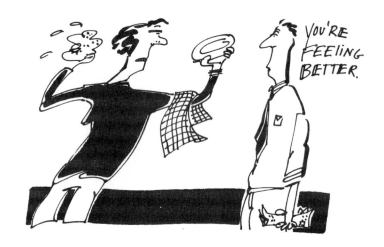

Friends and relatives are quite likely to become frustrated and angry when their offers of help are turned down by the depressed person. Nothing they do or say seems to make any difference. It can be very disheartening and eventually they will give up.

It is particularly distressing for children to see a parent or step-parent in such a debilitated state. They will need convincing that it is only temporary, like a broken limb. The fact that they cannot see the part that hurts doesn't mean it is not there.

If the children keep up their own hobbies, interests and friendships, these will cushion them against the difficulty of living with a depressed parent.

You also have a responsibility (if that is not too strong a word) to stay healthy and on top of the situation. It is not easy to keep things going. You will often get tired, physically, mentally and emotionally.

Sleep can become a problem for you if your partner's sleep pattern has changed. You need your rest. The solution might be as simple as asking your partner to go quietly into another room when he cannot sleep, make himself a cup of tea, or put on some music without disturbing the rest of the household. Or you could ask your GP for something to help you sleep, although tranquillisers should only be used as a last resort. There are herbal remedies on the market that are non-habit-forming and these can be bought over the counter.

No sex please, we're depressed

There are noticeable changes in someone when they are depressed. Their essential personality has temporarily withdrawn. They have lost their sense of humour, they have probably lost weight, and lost interest in sex.

At the onset of the illness, or in mild cases, sex is beneficial and therapeutic. Lovemaking should be an intimate, caring act that offers your partner the reassurance of your love.

When the depression really takes hold, all the pleasures of life, including sex, mean little or nothing at all. There may also be side-effects from the medication which decrease the libido. Your partner's withdrawal from sex is not directed at you, so don't take umbrage and think you have lost your sex appeal. It must not affect your relationship. To make love requires mental and physical energy, which a depressed person does not have. Also, you need to like yourself, to be happy with your body and your own sexuality. This too, is missing.

Unfortunately it can be a bit of a vicious circle. When a man is depressed he finds it difficult to get and sustain an erection. Because of this he feels less of a man and this increases his anxiety. Assure him that it doesn't make any difference to your relationship. You can still be intimate and loving, can still hug and caress. On no account reject him because he has 'gone off it', even if you are extremely hot-blooded! He will make up for it later on.

When a woman is depressed, she may submit to please her partner, but she is more likely to show lack of interest. She may see herself as physically unlovable and will need lots of reassurance that this is not so. Constant reassurance is important for your partner's self-esteem and in the long run, for your relationship.

How depression can affect different members of the family

If a person is in full-time work, the first effects of the illness might be put down to tiredness or working too hard. At work, lethargy and lack of concentration will result in problems, but colleagues and bosses will put it down to stress or the need for a holiday.

Gradually he or she will do less and less in the evenings and at weekends. It could be that at this stage a holiday would bring the person out of their depression, get them away from whatever is causing the stress. It is easier to see what is wrong from a distance and do something about it. At this stage it would be beneficial to have talking treatment.

Failing this, a GP might prescribe antidepressants to lift the mood sufficiently so that he or she can sort out their problems.

Being an emotional illness it is not always seen as something a man should suffer from. It is a 'wimp's' illness. His image of himself will take something of a knock. If the illness develops into something worse and his wife has to take the initiative in decision-making and financial matters, she should take care not to make an issue out of this role reversal, if it is such. It could damage his self-respect.

In the case of a depressed woman in a full-time job, much of the above applies. Where a woman is working part-time, or at home, her partner will need to rely on family and friends to keep the home running smoothly, as well as taking over her tasks. They may have friends with children the same age who would be willing to take the children for a few hours after school or playgroup. A husband might take time off, though going to work will help him to keep his own life as normal as possible. (The same goes for the mother, of course, when it is her partner who is ill.) He can then face the situation fresh each evening.

He should explain to the children that their mother is ill but that she will get better, and most importantly she still loves them.

When the mother is single or divorced, or in a situation where it is not suitable for the father to look after the children and there are no relatives able to do so, the social services will find temporary foster parents. As far as possible a good relationship is built up between the foster mother and the natural mother.

When a child or teenager is depressed, they express their unhappiness through their behaviour. Many adolescents suffer from bouts of depression. They are unsure of themselves, their emotions are wreaking havoc and there are additional pressures on them to 'achieve' at school or college.

Once you have made sure that it is not the sulks, you should get professional help. This is because you are emotionally involved and probably too close to see what is making them ill.

Don't be too proud to get help from your GP or a child guidance clinic. It does not mean you have

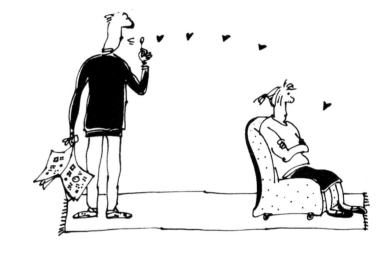

failed as a parent. On the contrary, as a caring parent you are doing the best for your child. Keep on loving them unconditionally. Hug and kiss them and offer encouragement and praise. Tell them you want to understand and help and that they must not be frightened, they will get better. Help their friends to understand the illness, too, and support them.

Parents or grandparents may become depressed on retirement. They imagine that they are no longer needed or useful. As they age, neither their eyesight nor hearing are what they used to be, nor are they as physically fit and able as they would like to be. Friends and acquaintances die and this can make them feel increasingly lonely.

When they become depressed, they show signs of confusion, forgetfulness and possibly incontinence. A grandparent who is well and cheerful is welcome in the family circle, but one who is depressed can put a great strain on the family.

It is a difficult age group to treat, because older people are less likely to complain of depression, not wanting to 'make a fuss'. Instead, they may complain of physical, bodily symptoms, which they feel are more acceptable to a doctor than an emotional complaint. When you realise an elderly relative is depressed, encourage them to seek professional help.

Their GP may suggest a short stay in hospital to help lift them out of the depression, but the great majority of older people are treated in their own homes.

Additional interests outside the home could help, once the depression starts to lift. Adult education classes have a wide variety of subjects on offer. Voluntary and charity work are another option, and some firms have a policy of taking over sixties onto their staff.

A retired person has the life experience and the freedom to help others. Retirement is a great opportunity to try things.

Explaining to others

There is a stigma attached to mental and emotional illnesses. Depression is often thought of as not being a 'proper' illness. The phrase 'nervous breakdown' is more acceptable than depression. People are frightened of things they don't understand. In 1992 a five-year campaign on depression was launched by the Royal College of Psychiatrists in association with the Royal College of General Practitioners. This aimed to emphasise that depression is common, recognisable and treatable.

As a carer you are in a position to help expel the myths surrounding mental illness. Your attitude can quell the anxieties of others. By now you will have gathered some facts about depression:

- it is temporary, the patient will recover
- it is a clinically diagnosed and common illness
- it can affect anyone of any age
- it can be treated
- it is not a weakness of character or a mood
- it is not 'insanity'
- the sufferer is not to blame for their condition
- it is an emotional disorder that can be as painful as a physical one
- it is usually brought on by one or more stress factors.

Accepting and explaining these facts to others and displaying both a caring and a positive attitude towards the sufferer will go a long way towards dispelling others' fears about depression.

For a long time I covered up for Peter's illness. Guilt and shame were part of this reluctance. But the more I learned about depression, the more I accepted it as a common illness and when I opened up at last and explained it to others it was like a weight being lifted from me.

Replacing negatives with positives

Time can drag endlessly when you are living with a depressed person. You find that you are thankful to get through each day. You can only live one day at a time, so tell yourself that it is one more 'bad' day behind you, another day nearer to the end of the illness.

Your depressed partner may be unable to count his blessings, but you certainly can. You'd be surprised how many you can come up with.

- Take time each day to look at or listen to something beautiful. Let it absorb you totally, take over your mind.
- Read for relaxation and escapism.
- Find helpful texts and passages that will give you moral and spiritual support. Share them with your partner.
- Bombard him with a constant repetition of positive thoughts, planting them in his subconscious.

I lost count of the times I repeated the words 'You *will* get better'. Sometimes I think it must have sounded more like a threat!

You loved him when he was strong and well. The challenge is to love him while he is weak and

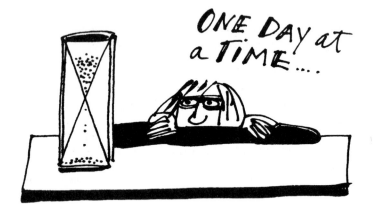

ONE DAY at a TIME....

debilitated. Even when you are exasperated and short of patience you have to show you care.

Let him know all the things you like about him (the well person, that is). Write out a list of his good and admirable qualities. Remember how you felt about him at the beginning of your relationship. Make sure he is not excluded from the family circle. Give him hope and optimism. Be gentle. Be kind.

Prayer support

Perhaps you do not pray. Maybe you think it does not work, you do not belong to any church, temple, synagogue or other place of worship, or somewhere along the line you have given-up believing for one reason or another.

It is often in times of crisis that we come back to prayer, although we may not be willing to admit this to others. Even if you are not at home with prayer – give it a try. Your depressed partner or friend is unable to pray for himself. Many religious people temporarily lose their faith when they are ill. They feel worthless and they may think that God has abandoned them. So,

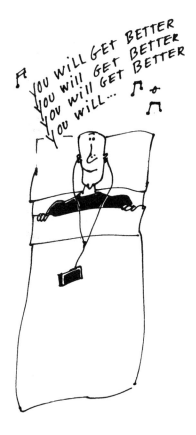

you have to do the praying for your partner – and with him. It is very difficult if you have never prayed in front of someone before, you will be self-conscious at first. It does not matter, take a deep breath before you start. It gets easier and it works.

As a carer you are already being used by God. He uses you through your patience and your caring to reach out to the depressive in a way that will last long after the illness has gone. He reaches through you to love and heal.

Prayer itself need not be confined to a set time each day, it is something you can do anywhere at any time. Begin by thanking God. Think of all you can give thanks for. A new day with new opportunities. Your health and strength, family, friends. Anything and everything. By starting with thanksgiving you have set yourself the right attitude of mind and lifted yourself up mentally and emotionally. It is a very positive thing to do.

It also makes it easier to ask God for His help in your present situation and His support in the future.

I can, of course, only speak from my own experience here, but my faith was of vital importance in helping me through.

4   Coping with your own feelings

We are emotional beings. Every single day emotions enter our lives. They are expressed in a variety of feelings – joy, sorrow, love, anger, excitement, hope.

A great deal of our behaviour is derived from emotion. It motivates us. It also causes physical changes in us. We tremble and turn pale with fright. We blush with pleasure or embarrassment. Our heart beats faster with excitement or fear. We laugh when we are amused or happy and cry when we are sad.

Emotion is an outward expression of something that is going on inside. Without emotions our lives would be flat and colourless.

Bewilderment and sympathy

At the beginning, you probably thought your partner was off-colour or going down with something. In fact, he was, although not quite in the way you had imagined. When the low mood persisted, you realised that it was not a normal everyday depression. Something more deep-seated was making him ill.

Your first reaction would have been sympathy, which is certainly what he needed. The closer you are to a person, the harder it is to watch them suffer. When you found yourself unable to talk him out of it, or find a reason for it, you became anxious and bewildered. Even where there is a reason, a bereavement or job loss, perhaps, your assurances made no difference.

At a stage when the depression was going from mild to more severe, you probably realised that your life was about to be turned upside-down and that there was nothing you could do to prevent it.

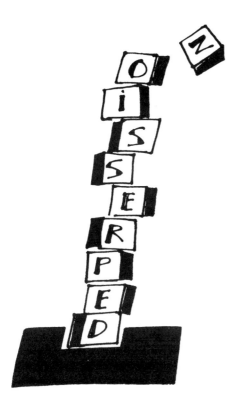

Guilt

The changes happen as he withdraws into himself. You cannot stir him out of his apathy for any length of time, or stimulate his interest in anything. He responds less and less and this can be very frustrating. You question yourself. Does my love mean nothing? Why was I unable to prevent the illness in the first place? Why didn't I see it coming? Is it my fault?

What may be an emotive issue to you is not the same for the depressed person. The illness makes him unable to feel or accept pleasure and love, on the surface at any rate. His illness could be seen as a sort of virus, a disease against which he has not been immunised. He must wait until it is worked out of his system.

A clinical depression will run its course in about 18 months. During much of that time the patient will be recovering and able to function almost normally. He will have some 'down' days but these will be manageable.

Guilt and self-blame are common emotions when you live with someone who is depressed. (My love hasn't helped him, therefore I don't love him enough.) When he appears to reject you, you think it is your fault. What did you do wrong? You have failed him.

Going through recent events in your mind you wonder whether you might have been responsible in any way for his depression. He has not been able to talk things out with you, so perhaps the cause lies in your relationship. You feel guilty and at the same time irritated at being made to feel guilty.

There are two obvious answers. Either the depression has nothing to do with you, or it *has*.

Certainly I felt I was very much to blame. I had made Peter leave his home for a totally different way of life when he was already vulnerable and in need of bereavement counselling.

Although it is true that relationship problems can trigger off depression it is sometimes not obvious, possibly because the couple are so close, or because one of them has pushed down the feelings of anger, inadequacy or hurt.

It may be possible to work out your own answer to your partner's problem, perhaps with help from an uninvolved friend. If all is well in your relationship, stop blaming yourself. If not, you need help in sorting it out, with counselling or family therapy. You cannot undo the past but you can make an effort to improve the future.

Living with a stranger

The symptoms of depression are easier to read about than to live with. The qualities that attracted you to your partner originally are no longer there. Gone is the cheerful, dynamic, caring person. In his place is an intruder!

There are physical changes as well as emotional ones. He is 'not himself', he looks ill. He may display tenseness, agitation and trembling. His breath may not be as sweet as a summer's day. When you embrace, he has lost so much weight that you can feel bones sticking out where you never felt them before.

He does, in fact, appear to be a different person altogether, physically, mentally and emotionally.

The insecurity of being without your supportive partner, plus the loneliness this brings, can be discouraging. How long, you wonder, will you manage without him.

Have faith in yourself, you will manage. We are all capable of a great deal more than we give ourselves credit for. A parent whose child had been trapped underneath a car unhesitatingly lifted up the front of the car so that he could be pulled clear. You often find unsuspected strength and ability in challenging circumstances.

Above all, even though you hate what the illness has done to him, let him know that you love him anyway.

Covering up

Reluctance to tell others what is happening to your partner or relative is understandable, especially if you have never experienced a depressive illness before. It may even be that you don't want to worry others, for example elderly parents.

Usually, though, you hide it from them because of the stigma still attached to mental illness. Another reason for keeping them at arm's length is the embarrassment you think will be felt when family, friends or colleagues visit. The person you love and were so proud of sits there full of self-pity, looking pathetic.

The sufferer needs his friends and family, needs to know he is not being avoided and hidden away, needs to know that people care. The taboos connected with psychiatric illness arise out of ignorance. Your

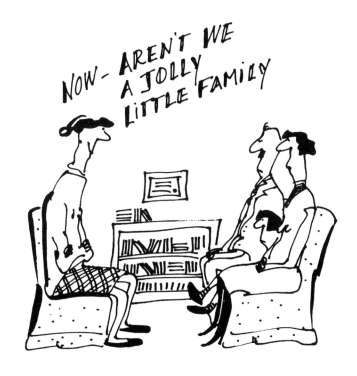

attitude, as suggested earlier, should be a positive one. Reread the list of facts about depression and reinforce your own feelings.

Mental distress is such a common problem that most people will know someone who has been treated for it. Show sympathy and understanding towards the depressive and others will take the cue. Who knows, they are probably telling themselves, 'There, but for the Grace of God, go I'.

It's a cop-out

Anger is an emotion many of us try to suppress because it is considered antisocial, a lack of self-control. When we are angry with a depressed partner we feel ashamed.

Our anger grows out of irritation and exasperation. There is resentment too. You feel he isn't trying to help himself – even though you know he can't and you are being irrational.

You are angry because you have been placed in a situation which has disrupted your life. You feel let down. You ask yourself, how could he do this to you? Where is his backbone? He has deserted you and left you to fend for yourself.

'He's not the man I married – he's cracked up, let us down and I resent it!'

Totally irrational, but also very human. You get angry with his constant repetition of negative thoughts, which are all exaggerations, if not completely untrue. He says he is worthless, better off dead. You can't convince him he's wrong. He just sits there completely self-absorbed, ignoring you. He has opted out. Your patience is frayed at the edges. In fact, you don't feel in the least bit tender and loving.

In the circumstances it is natural to be angry. The difficult part is not to do it in his presence. Go for a long walk and be angry where it can't hurt or offend anyone. Write out your angry feelings. Thump your pillow. Cry it out of your system. Do some hard physical exercise and wear yourself out. Just make sure that you do not say anything you will regret later. Words spoken in the heat of the moment when you are emotionally upset can do lasting damage.

Be angry at the illness, not its victim. It will need teeth-gritting determination. Tell yourself you will *not* let it beat you, you are damned if you will!

Something else which you might experience is an attack of the night panics: that sinking feeling in the pit of your stomach, quickened heartbeat and anxious thoughts in the early hours of the morning. Although it does pass, it can be frightening at the time. One way to get through it is to repeat a positive statement over and over again. Things look better in the morning, and you will be able to cope with the demands made on you for a little while longer.

Exhaustion

Stress is exhausting. You are under stress when you are with someone who is depressed. They sap your energy. The closer the relationship, the more emotionally exhausting it is for you.

'I can't go on like this much longer.' No matter how much patience and energy you possess there will be times when you are worn out, depleted. A sort of love-worn-thin, when you have reached the end of your resources – or think you have.

It may not take much to restore you. A good night's sleep, an outing with friends or even a sympathetic ear can help. You must take care not to let yourself get run down too far, to the point of hopelessness and despair. It is no use you *both* being depressed. So, selfish though it may sound, it is important for you to keep going.

I was lucky in that our children were old enough to understand what was happening and able to retain their sense of humour throughout. The one time I felt really low, they said 'Not you, too, Mum', and that brought me up sharply.

You should try and remove yourself from the situation temporarily. A short period every day may be enough to recharge your batteries. If you are in need of a longer break your GP or social worker may be able to arrange for the patient to stay in hospital while you are away.

It is vital to keep your sense of humour alive and kicking. Spend time with people who can cheer you up, members of your family and circle of friends who can see the funny side of life. Humour helps you to keep life events in proportion. Do relaxing things together. See a film or play. Go to a concert. Take up a new hobby or learn a new skill, something totally absorbing. Go dancing. Release your pent-up emotions in the best way you can. This is not being callous, it is survival.

When you are with the patient, keep yourself busy and try to switch off from his misery if you can. Don't let it get you down. Don't measure time, wondering when you will see the light at the end of the tunnel. Each person is different. Each depression is different.

Get him to talk about something other than himself, it will help him out of his negative thought pattern. Visitors can often help here, bringing in fresh news and views.

All the emotions you experience, bewilderment, sympathy, anger, guilt, anxiety, loneliness and anger, are normal human reactions to a stressful situation. A carer is in a vulnerable situation, so there is no shame in expressing feelings rather than bottling then up and giving yourself an ulcer.

Having said that, take care that your feelings do not get exaggerated or out of hand. Someone who is depressed needs loving support, not anger or sadness. It is difficult concealing your 'bad' feelings from him, that is why you need to get away when you can.

When you are really low and feeling sorry for yourself, try to imagine life without your partner or relative. Weigh up the pros and cons. It sounds heartless, but it is a worthwhile exercise and will give you renewed determination to see them restored to health. Looking back through a family photo album with its happy memories may help.

Hang on to the little things which enhance daily life. Open your eyes to the beauty around you and indulge your senses.

Remember, too, that you already have a source of strength to draw from daily. Someone who is willing to take over when you can no longer cope. Nothing that happens to you cannot be shared with God. He is on your side even in the worst circumstances. He can help.

5 Handing over

Sometimes depression reaches a stage where it simply cannot be handled at home, even by the most loving and patient of families. It has gone so deep that the sufferer is no longer aware of what they are doing or saying. It is time to get professional help and call the doctor.

Our Silver Wedding Anniversary is a day imprinted on my memory. Peter had been growing increasingly ill, was neither resting nor eating and had lost an enormous amount of weight. He had even tried to throw himself out of the landing window. He was sure he was dying. There was no choice left, and with the GP, psychiatrist, social worker and psychiatric nurse crammed into our small living room, he was put 'on section'.

How does it feel when someone you love has to go into a psychiatric hospital?

In a recent report arising out of a MIND public meeting on 'The first 24 hours after admission into a psychiatric hospital', the views of users, staff and relatives were put forward. It was found that relatives were affected as much as those who were receiving psychiatric care. Guilt, relief, uncertainty and fear were among the mixed feelings experienced. Guilt – was it the carer's fault? Relief at handing over the responsibility and not having to cope any longer. Uncertainty as to the future and fear of what family and friends might think. There must also be a great deal of uncertainty about what happens on first admission to a psychiatric hospital.

Every patient who is admitted to hospital has a primary, or named nurse. This nurse will have a small group of patients who are her particular concern, and with whom she or he is in daily contact. When they are off duty, other nurses from the same team will look after those patients. The relationship between primary nurse and patient is important. In fact, if for any reason the patient does not feel comfortable with the primary nurse, they can ask for another of the nurses in that team.

On admission, the patient and his relatives will be shown into an admission room where the procedure is explained and various forms signed. There is a welcome pack, which will explain how the ward is run: times of meals, fire drill, ward layout, laundry facilities, care of valuables, visiting hours, etc.

Also included in the welcome pack are the initial care plan, the names of the consultant psychiatrist, his/her registrar, the ward manager and the primary nurse.

The team of carers, known as the multi-disciplinary team, also includes social workers, physiotherapists, occupational therapists, art therapists, community psychiatric workers and the ward nurses who assist in caring for your relative. He will meet most of these during his stay, depending on his own particular needs.

Patients who are detained on a section will have their rights explained to them within 24 hours. Under the Mental Health Act 1983, someone may be compulsorily detained in hospital for their own health or safety and the safety of others. This is only used as a last resort. On admission some depressed patients are too agitated, confused or suicidal to take anything in. The presence of the carer is important here.

There is a Patient's Charter displayed prominently on the wall of the ward explaining a patient's rights.

If they appear to be suicidal or are in any way at risk, they may be put on level 1 observation. This means that they are accompanied by a nurse 24 hours a day. Level 2 observation means that a nurse will check their whereabouts every 15 minutes. These observations are reassessed daily by the doctor.

Once the patient has been admitted, they are shown round the ward and the ward policy explained to them. They are taken to their room or dormitory to unpack, while a nurse fills in a property form with them.

Treatments

Antidepressant drugs

Most severe cases of depression require treatment with antidepressant drugs. These affect the chemicals in the brain which are associated with depression. They are not addictive. Some may cause side-effects such as drowsiness, shaky hands or a dry mouth. Others require a controlled diet which does not include such things as cheese, Marmite and broad beans. Some drugs have to be taken for about two weeks before results are noticed, but they are effective and in about 70% of cases the patient responds to the treatment. They must continue with the medication for several weeks or even months after the depression has lifted, and taken off it gradually on the doctor's guidance.

While the antidepressants do not take away the cause of the illness they do relieve the symptoms, enabling the patient to deal with the problems which caused the depression.

Electroconvulsive therapy

Electroconvulsive therapy (ECT) is prescribed for certain patients as a way of lifting them out of a deep depression when antidepressants are not enough, or when the pain of depression is so great that the patient is at risk of suicide.

ECT is a controversial treatment because in the past it was often used indiscriminately. Nowadays it is safe, painless and quick. It is given under strict medical supervision. The treatment is given two or three times a week over a limited period. Usually six treatments are sufficient, and dramatic improvements can be seen sometimes after only two. The patient is given a light anaesthetic and muscle relaxant before a controlled electric current is passed through the brain. The patient may wake with a slight headache or a feeling of confusion and muddle-headedness, but this soon wears off.

There is now a greater understanding of how ECT works. The seizure produces a chemical change in the neurotransmitter system in the brain. There may be a temporary, mild, memory loss, which in some cases lasts up to two weeks or longer, but this may be due to the depression itself and not the ECT.

Therapies

Although drugs help lift a depressive mood by altering the balance of chemicals in the brain, they do not deal with the problems that brought on the depression in the first place. Therapists have different methods of helping a patient.

The ward may have its own programme of patients' activities, which help the patient by occupying them, helping them relax and building up their confidence and self-esteem. Other members of the care team, the art therapists, occupational therapists and physiotherapists are on hand. Representatives from the Citizens' Advice Bureau and the substance misuse team visit weekly. Anxiety management and assertiveness groups are often available, if not on the ward, then in the day centre attached to the hospital.

Talking treatments such as bereavement counselling and family counselling may be available. A patient may be referred to a psychologist or psycho-therapist for treatment. In psychotherapy the doctor tries to understand childhood traumas that have made the patient vulnerable to depression, or other events or relationships which could have led up to it. The type of treatment your relative undergoes is worked out by their support team and discussed during their care plan assessment.

Patients are often able to help each other. They share the experience of mental distress and those who are on the path to recovery offer support, hope and encouragement to others. Once your relative starts to improve he will be given home leave, perhaps for a day, then a weekend. Gradually this is lengthened until he is ready for discharge.

6   Making progress together

At last you know things are looking up. Your partner is home on leave from hospital and you can see the improvement in him. In fact, in some cases the patient is so delighted that the black cloud of depression has lifted that he becomes extremely elated. He may go on a shopping spree or phone family and friends to tell them how marvellous he feels. Peter sent our phone bill soaring with several calls to South Africa to tell people he was better!

Beware! It is like a roller coaster, he will come down from those dizzy heights. When he does it will be a shook to him, an unwelcome, unexpected and, he thinks, insurmountable setback. It isn't. It is in the nature of things, one of the tricks that depression plays – four steps forward and one step back. The mood swings level off over a period of time. However, when he does come down off a 'high', some of the old feelings of fear and failure return.

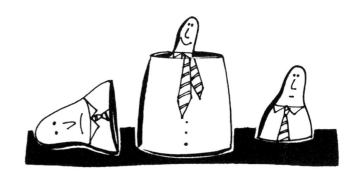

It is only temporary, though at this stage he may well be saying 'I'll never get better'. He will. Keep reassuring him that this is part of depression and it will pass. His mood will fluctuate. When it goes up again it will not be as high, or as low when it dips. He may be desperately disappointed when he goes down, feeling that he cannot trust or control his mood.

It might be helpful for him to draw a graph so that he is able to see the gradual improvement as it happens, feel encouraged by it, and shake off the bad days more easily. Just knowing he will have a few downs will help him ride them out. Each step on the graph is progress on the road to recovery – highs and lows. Each time he comes out of a dip he is nearer the end of his illness.

When his mood is stabilised, it is a good idea to look at your lifestyle and see if any changes can be made that will lessen the stress.

- Cut out things you can do without in order to save money
- Duties that can be delegated to others
- Discuss his problems one at a time, not all together

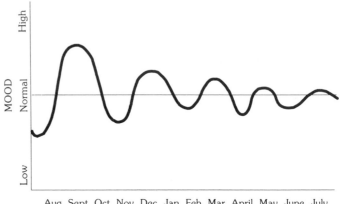

(The dip between April and May occurred after the patient had attended a three-day users' conference. He had enjoyed it so much that he felt flat afterwards.)

- Go over the reasons for his illness and see whether they are still valid.

This is the stage where further counselling might be necessary. If he spent time in hospital his multi-disciplinary team will have given him a care plan assessment. There is a network of groups in the community that can provide back-up.

Day hospitals

Day hospitals are an alternative to in-patient care. They provide group therapies and intensive support for out-patients, with such things as anxiety management, play-reading, relaxation, circuit-training (exercises in the gym) and art and crafts. Patients are referred to day hospitals by their nursing team, or a CPN or doctor.

Drop-in centres

Drop-in centres offer social contact with people who have similar problems. There may be a user group in your area. Though each group has slightly different aims and objectives they all identify the needs of the user.

Getting back to work

These in turn will link up to other areas of help: the Job Club, the Training and Enterprise Council, psychometric tests, and any free training that is available in the area. Adult education courses are widespread and voluntary workers are always in demand to teach basic skills. This can be an enormous confidence booster.

Recuperation period

The main thing during this recuperation period is that he does not sit back feeling sorry for himself. Encourage him to keep a diary in which to express his feelings and mood but also to note the positive things he has accomplished each day. This will reinforce his feelings of self-worth. Writing things out of your system can be very therapeutic. Many patients are encouraged to write their life story starting with their very first memories.

Unwind together, listening to music, or watching sport, whatever your favourite method of relaxing involves. Enjoy yourselves together and with friends.

Laughter is renowned as a therapy. There is even a NHS Laughter Clinic in Birmingham. (Laughter being taken seriously?) Laughing relaxes the body by reducing muscle tension and lowering blood pressure. It stimulates the brain to release chemicals called endorphins which not only relieve pain but are thought to influence the way we react to stress and make us feel good. Regular exercise has a similar effect.

Listening to relaxation tapes can be very beneficial. There is a good selection on the market. Let him take things at a gentle pace and build on it gradually. Some days he may not want to do much. It does not matter.

Tomorrow will be better. Soon he will be driving a car again, getting back to his hobbies, thinking about going back to work or job hunting.

The big turning point is when he is ready to make love again. It is more than just resuming your sex life, it is his announcement that he is better. Are you ready or is he still a stranger?

7   Your role as carer

By now you will understand how important your role is in your partner's recovery.

You have helped him through the worst of the illness, supporting him mentally, physically, emotionally, spiritually and probably financially. The fact that you have been there, loving him, often having to hide your frustration and exasperation, has meant a lot to him.

You have promoted a positive attitude, repeating 'You *will* get better' endlessly. You have coped with everyday living, helping family and friends to understand what was happening and above all tried to remain cheerful and bright when you felt rotten.

You have learned enough about depression to recognise and combat any future bouts, though this is probably unnecessary if the follow-up counselling has sorted out his problems, or alternatively, helped him to see them in a different light.

Through love, enormous effort and grim determination you have helped your partner and yourself through a crisis point in the relationship and you are stronger for having done so. You will find that your relationship has improved – you know so much more about each other now, your hopes and dreams as well as your fears. You have reached greater understanding, developed a compassion which will be tested again and again in the future as you come across others who need the encouragement and advice that you can now offer. Your life has been enriched.

See yourself as channelling love and healing and watch the results. You could surprise yourself!

Appendix: Where to go for help

There are a lot of things that can be done to help people who suffer from depression. If you think you may be depressed, then it can be helpful to talk to someone about how you are feeling. Do not bottle things up. Sharing problems with someone can help you to work out new solutions and discover new ways of coping.

However, if these feelings persist and start affecting your life, it is important to go and see your family doctor. The doctor may suggest some form of talking treatment, antidepressant tablets or both. Antidepressants are not tranquillisers and are therefore not addictive, although they may help you feel less anxious and agitated. They can take up to three weeks before your mood improves and like all medicines, they do have some side-effects. It is necessary for most people to continue taking them for around six months. The main groups of antidepressants are the tricyclics, the monoamine oxidase inhibitors (MAOIs) and the selective serotonin reuptake inhibitors (SSRIs). Ask your GP for details.

When antidepressants do not work or your family doctor is concerned about other underlying problems, you may be referred to your local mental health service. You are likely to be referred to a psychiatrist for more specialised help; however, it could also be a psychologist, CPN or social worker.

Very severely depressed people, who are actively suicidal, have stopped eating or drinking, and are even deluded, are usually unfit for treatment with antidepressants at home and may need to be referred to hospital. ECT is a physical treatment which can be used in very severe cases of depressive illness. In suitably selected cases, this treatment successfully relieves the terrible suffering which depression inflicts. The Royal College of Psychiatrists has produced a factsheet 'ECT: What You Need to Know', which can answer many of your fears about this treatment.

Self-help/support groups can be very helpful too. These groups offer you the chance to meet other people who have experienced depression, but in a small and informal gathering. It is not just a listening ear but a sharing experience, suggesting ways of coping and receiving encouragement, reassurance and support that you are not alone. (Self-help should not be confused with group therapy or encounter groups.)

More and more GPs are now employing counsellors in their practices, so do not forget to ask. Counselling is concerned with problem-solving and can reassure, restore a sense of proportion, and encourage a positive and practical approach to coping with your feelings and life in general. It is important that your counsellor is professionally trained.

In order to see a qualified psychotherapist you will need to ask your GP to refer you. It is important that a psychotherapist has a recognised qualification. You should not be afraid to shop around for someone who suits your needs. There are a number of psychological treatments available. Psychotherapy aims to discover the causes of the depression which the sufferer cannot at that time face. Within psychotherapy, there are a number of different schools, but what they all have in common is that they are all talking treatments. For instance, *psychodynamic psychotherapy* focuses on the feelings you have about other people, especially family and people close to you, and helps you to see how past experiences affect your life now. *Behavioural psychotherapy* aims, however, to change patterns of behaviour more directly. *Cognitive therapy* deals with the negative feelings which are often associated with depression. It looks at the 'here and now' issues rather than things of the past and helps you to learn new methods of coping and problem-solving that can be used for the rest of your life. *Family and marital therapy* deals with people's problems which are not often theirs alone but are the result of relationship problems in marriage, partnership or family.

Finally, there are a number of organisations which can help you, including the Samaritans, MIND and Relate, which are mentioned at the back of this book. For some people, alternative or complementary therapies such as homeopathy, acupuncture and even pet therapy may help where conventional treatments have not. Mild forms of exercise has also been shown to have helped people with less severe depression.

Deborah Hart,
Head of External Affairs, Royal College of Psychiatrists

Helpful addresses

Association for Postnatal Illness (APNI)
Can put you in touch with other mothers who have come through postnatal depression.

Jerdan Place, Fulham, London SW6 1BE
Tel: 0171 386 086825

The British Association for Counselling
Will provide a list of nationwide counsellors.

1 Regent Place, Warwick Street, Rugby, Warwickshire CV21 2PJ
Tel: 01788 578328

Carers' National Association
Provides information and advice for carers. Your local branch may run a carers' self-support group.

20–25 Glasshouse Yard, London EC1A 4JS
Tel: 0171 490 8818

Cruse Bereavement Care
Provides help and information for those who have been bereaved.

Cruse House, 126 Sheen Road, Richmond, Surrey TW9 IUR
Tel: 0181 332 7227 (bereavement line)
     0181 940 4818 (administration)

Depressives Anonymous (Fellowship of)
Organisation run as a source of support for sufferers, complementary to professional care.

36 Chestnut Avenue, Beverley, East Yorkshire HU17 9QU
Tel: 01482 860619

Depression Alliance
Information, support and understanding for people who suffer with depression and for relatives who want to help.

35 Westminster Bridge Road, London SE1 7QB
Tel: 0171 633 9929 (answerphone)

Department of Social Security Freeline
Offers advice and information on how to claim benefits.

Tel: 0800 666555

The Manic Depression Fellowship
Network of local self-help groups for sufferers and their families.

8–10 High Street, Kingston upon Thames, Surrey KT1 1EY
Tel: 0181 974 6550

MIND (National Association for Mental Health)
Publications and advice leaflets on mental health problems.

Granta, 15–19 Broadway, Stratford, London E15 4BQ
Tel: 0181 519 2122 (or your local branch)

National Association for Premenstrual Syndrome

Information line: 01732 741709

Relate
Marriage and relationship problems (formerly Marriage Guidance Council).

Herbert Grey College, Little Church Street, Rugby CV21 3AP
Tel: 01788 573241 (or your local branch)

Royal College of Psychiatrists
Patient information on common mental health problem treatments.

17 Belgrave Square, London SW1X 8PG
Tel: 0171 235 2351

The Samaritans
National organisation offering support to those in distress who feel suicidal or despairing and need someone to talk to. The Samaritans have 204 branches around the country open 24 hours a day, every day of the year. The telephone number of your local branch can be found in the telephone directory.

10 The Grove, Slough SL1 1QP
Tel: 0345 909090 (national helpline)
     01753 532713 (administration)

UK Council for Psychotherapy (UKCP)
Provides information on how to access appropriately qualified psychotherapists.

Regent's College, Inner Circle, Regent's Park, London NW1 4NS
Tel: 0171 487 7554

Index